The No-No

MENOPAUSAL

WEIGHT LOSS

Guide

Make it Happen by Following these Simple,
Effective, and safe Strategies.

Davina Sutton

© Copyright 2022 by Davina Sutton - All rights reserved.

The content contained within this book may not be reproduced, duplicated or transmitted without direct written permission from the author or the publisher.
Under no circumstances will any blame or legal responsibility be held against the publisher, or author, for any damages, reparation, or monetary loss due to the information contained within this book, either direct or indirectly.

Legal Notice:

This book is copyright protected. This book is only for personal use. You cannot amend, distribute, sell, use, quote or paraphrase any part or the content within this book, without the consent of the author or publisher.

Disclaimer Notice:

Please note the information contained within this document is for educational and entertainment purposes only. All effort has been executed to present accurate, up to date, reliable, complete information. No warranties of any kind are declared or implied. Readers acknowledge that the author is not engaged in the rendering of legal, financial, medical or professional advice. The content within this book has been derived from various sources. Please consult a licensed professional before attempting any techniques outlined in this book.

By reading this document, the reader agrees that under no circumstances is the author responsible for any losses, direct or indirect, that are incurred as a result of the use of the information contained within this document, including ,but not limited to, errors, omissions or inaccuracies.

TABLE OF CONTENTS

INTRODUCTION

Significant changes occur with menopause. Not only do your periods finally stop, but you also lose the ability to become pregnant. The reason for this is that your body no longer produces the quantities of estrogen and progesterone necessary for conception and reproduction.

It's important to realize that menopausal weight gain doesn't happen immediately. In other words, after your periods cease, you won't suddenly put on 10 pounds. The weight gain is more sluggish. According to a study, women may gain an average of 5 pounds during menopause. Women already overweight are more likely to put on weight at this time in their lives. Your risk of gaining weight can also be increased by other factors, including poor lifestyle choices.

When you consider menopause, you might immediately conjure up images of hot flashes and mood swings. While these symptoms are undoubtedly brought on by the decline in estrogen and progesterone that occurs throughout menopause, maintaining a healthy body weight over a lifetime can be simpler if you learn how to prevent weight gain today.

CHAPTER 1: UNDERSTANDING MENOPAUSE

What is menopause?

The definition of menopause is the condition of not having menstrual periods for a full year. The final menstrual period marks the end of the menopausal transition, which begins with variable menstrual cycle lengths. The phrase **"perimenopause"** refers to the period just preceding menopause. It is frequently used to describe the time leading up to menopause. Although it isn't a recognized medical term, it is occasionally employed to explain certain menopause transitional aspects in simple terms. The time period following menopause is referred to as **"postmenopausal"** as an adjective. Doctors may refer to a condition as occurring in "postmenopausal women," for instance. Menopausal women are those who have already experienced it.

Menopause is the period of a woman's life when her ovaries stop working. She is unable to become pregnant as a result. One of two female reproductive glands is the ovary, often known as the female gonad. One is located on either side of the uterus in the pelvis. The size and form of each ovary are comparable to those of an almond. The ovaries produce ova, which are eggs, as well as estrogen and other female hormones. A single ovary releases an egg once per monthly menstrual cycle. The Fallopian tube connects the ovary to the uterus where the egg develops.

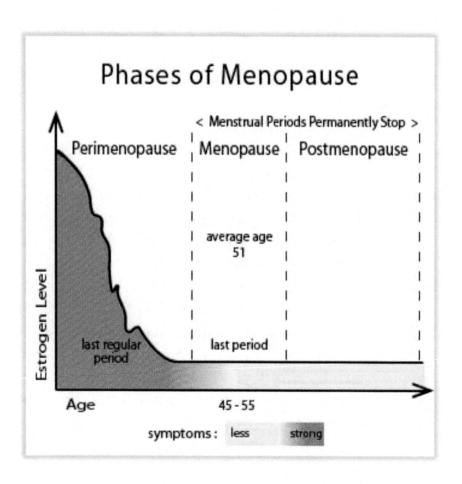

The primary source of female hormones, which regulate the growth of female body features including the breasts, body shape, and body hair, is the ovaries. The menstrual cycle and pregnancy are also controlled by hormones. The bone is also shielded by estrogen. As a result, if a woman's ovaries do not generate enough estrogen, she may develop osteoporosis (thinning of the bone) later in life.

What is the average age at which a woman experiences menopause?

Menopause typically occurs at 51 years of age. However, it is impossible to anticipate when a particular woman will go through menopause or start exhibiting signs of it. The age at which a woman begins menstruating is also unrelated to the age at which menopause first occurs. Menopause often occurs between the ages of 45 and 55 in women, but it can also start as early as the 30s or 40s or wait until a woman is 60. As a general "rule of thumb," women typically experience menopause at about the same age as their mothers. Menopausal symptoms and indications, such as anomalies in the menstrual cycle, can start up to ten years before the final menstrual period.

How long does menopause last?

Menopause, or the time when a woman's last period finishes, is a discrete moment in time rather than a process. Of course, until she has gone 12 months without a period, a woman won't be able to tell when that time point has come. On the other hand, menopause symptoms can start years before the transition to menopause and can last for a number of years thereafter.

❖ What are the symptoms and indicators of menopause?

It's crucial to keep in mind that every woman's experience is really unique. While some women may have few or no menopause symptoms, others may have several physical and psychological ones. Women experience a wide range of symptom intensity and breadth. Additionally, it's crucial to keep in mind that for some women, symptoms may come and go over a lengthy period of time. This is also quite individualized. Below, we go into more detail about these menopause and perimenopause symptoms.

1. Unusual vaginal bleeding

Women who are approaching menopause may experience irregular vaginal bleeding. Prior to menopause, some women experience only minor issues with irregular bleeding, while others experience erratic, heavy bleeding. Menstrual periods (menses) can come more frequently, which shortens the cycle, or they can spread out further and further apart, which lengthens the cycle before finishing. There is no "typical" pattern of bleeding during perimenopause, and individual women have different patterns. Women in perimenopause frequently experience their first period after spending several months without one. The time it takes for a woman to go through the menopausal transition is also not predetermined. Before menopause, a woman may experience years of irregular menstruation. To ensure that the irregular menses are caused by perimenopause and not as a sign of another medical issue, it is crucial to keep in mind that all women who experience irregular menstruation should be assessed by their doctor.

Due to irregular ovulation, the monthly irregularities that start in perimenopause are also linked to a decline in fertility. Perimenopausal women should still use contraception if they don't want to get pregnant because they can still become pregnant until they attain real menopause (a year without periods).

2. Severe hot flashes

Women going through menopause often have hot flashes. An all-over sensation of warmth known as a "hot flash" is often strongest in the head and chest. Perspiration may come after a hot flash, and it may be accompanied by flushing. Typically, hot flashes persist for about 30 to several minutes. Although the precise reason for hot flashes is unknown, they are probably caused by a mix of hormonal and metabolic changes brought on by low estrogen levels.

There is currently no way to anticipate the onset and duration of hot flashes. Approximately 40% of women who are routinely menstruating in their forties experience hot flashes; hence, they may start before the monthly irregularities that are a hallmark of menopause even happen. After five years, 80% of women will no longer experience hot flashes. Hot flashes can occasionally (in about 10% of women) linger for up to 10 years. Although the frequency of hot flashes tends to diminish over time, there is no way to anticipate when they will stop. Their severity may also fluctuate. The average woman who has hot flashes will do so for five years on average.

Night sweats can occasionally accompany hot flashes (episodes of drenching sweats at nighttime). This could cause waking up and having trouble falling asleep again, which would result in restless sleep and fatigue during the day.

3. Nighttime sweating

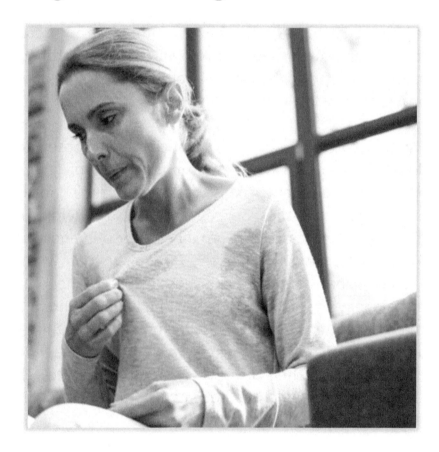

Hot flashes can occasionally be accompanied by night sweats, which are episodes of intense overnight sweating. This could cause waking up and trouble to fall asleep again, which would result in restless sleep and fatigue during the day.

4. Vaginal symptoms

As estrogen levels fall, the tissues lining the vagina become thinner, drier, and less elastic, which leads to vaginal discomfort. Vaginal dryness, itching, discomfort, and/or pain during sexual activity are possible symptoms. Additionally, vaginal alterations raise the risk of vaginal infections.

5. Urinary problems

Similar to the tissues of the vagina, the lining of the urethra (the transport tube leading from the bladder to discharge pee outside the body) likewise experiences changes with diminishing estrogen levels and becomes drier, thinner, and less elastic. This may result in a higher risk of urinary tract infection, a greater urge to urinate frequently, or urine leaks (urinary incontinence). A sudden, urgent urge to urinate can cause incontinence, as can straining while laughing, coughing, or moving heavy objects.

6. Mental and emotional symptoms

Many other mental (cognitive) and/or emotional symptoms, such as weariness, memory issues, impatience, and abrupt mood swings, are frequently reported by perimenopausal women. It might be challenging to pinpoint precisely which behavioral symptoms are caused by menopause's hormonal changes. For a variety of reasons, this area of research has been challenging.

It might be challenging for a woman to determine whether emotional or cognitive symptoms are related to menopause because they are so widespread. Having night sweats during perimenopause may also make you feel fatigued and worn out, which can affect your mood and your ability to think clearly. Last but not least, many women may be going through other life changes before or after menopause, like stressful life events, which can also result in emotional problems.

7. Other physical changes

Many women claim that menopause is accompanied by some degree of weight gain. Body fat may now be distributed differently, with more being stored around the waist and abdomen than the hips and thighs. Adult acne sufferers may notice changes in their skin's texture, including wrinkles, as well as an aggravation of their condition. Some women may notice hair growth on the chin, upper lip, chest, or belly because the body still produces trace amounts of the male hormone testosterone.

❖ What factors can result in early menopause?

The timing of menopause might be affected by specific medical and surgical issues.

Surgery to remove the ovaries

An ovulating woman who undergoes an oophorectomy will experience instantaneous menopause, often known as surgical menopause or induced menopause. There is no perimenopause in this situation, and a woman would typically suffer menopausal symptoms and signs after surgery. Women frequently report that the abrupt beginning of menopausal symptoms leads to particularly severe symptoms in cases of surgical menopause, but this is not always the case.

The removal of the uterus is frequently followed by the excision of the ovaries (hysterectomy). The remaining ovary or ovaries can still produce hormones normally if a hysterectomy is performed on a woman who has not yet achieved menopause without removing both ovaries. A hysterectomy prevents a woman from having periods, but the ovaries themselves can continue to generate hormones until menopause would normally starts to occur. Hot flashes and mood swings are two more menopause symptoms that a woman could encounter at this time. The cessation of menstruation would not then be linked to these symptoms. Another risk is that one to two years after the hysterectomy, premature ovarian failure will happen before the projected menopause time. A woman could or might not suffer menopausal symptoms if this occurs.

Chemotherapy and radiation therapy for cancer

If given to an ovulating woman, these cancer therapies (chemotherapy and/or radiation therapy) may cause menopause depending on the kind, location, and treatment of cancer. Menopause symptoms in this situation could appear months after the cancer therapy or they could start during the cancer therapy.

Premature ovarian failure

Menopause starting before the age of 40 is known as "premature ovarian failure. Approximately 1% of all women have this issue. Although the exact etiology of early ovarian failure is unknown, autoimmune disorders or inherited (genetic) factors may play a role.

FACTS ABOUT EARLY MENOPAUSE

Your period was thus missed. Or two. I'm too young for menopause, you tell yourself. Right? "
No, not always. 5% of women have early menopause between the ages of 40 and 45. Approximately 1% of women experience premature menopause, which occurs before age 40.

If you have gone a complete 12 months without having a period, you are considered to be in menopause. The female hormones required to maintain your monthly cycles and fertility, estrogen and progesterone, stop being produced by your ovaries at that time. Menopause typically starts at around age 51 for women. Many women will spend up to 40% of their lives in the postmenopausal stage as a result of longer life expectancies.

Some women experience an early onset of menopause as a result of life-saving procedures like surgery, chemotherapy, or radiation. Others may experience this alteration as a result of hereditary abnormalities, autoimmune diseases, or even unidentified causes.

Menopause symptoms can range from bothersome to dangerous and include hot flashes, sleep disturbances, dry eyes, and weight gain. However, if you are going through these things in your 20s, 30s, or early 40s, it could feel like you're aging faster than your pals and like you're becoming older overnight.

And here's the thing: When you start to enter premature or early menopause, there aren't usually obvious indicators. Who isn't moody? You might be one of them. The onset of heat flashes may or may not be imminent. You might not even be aware of how a hot flash feels. A hot flash is an abrupt sensation of warmth that travels throughout the body. It usually feels the strongest in the face, neck, and chest areas. Some ladies can experience a slight flushing. Other women wind up drenched in sweat and require bed linen changes.

What should you do in the absence of a large neon banner that reads "Welcome to Menopause"?

5 THINGS ABOUT EARLY MENOPAUSE YOU SHOULD KNOW

1. It's not too early to consult with your doctor. Make an appointment for an examination if your periods dramatically alter (become visibly longer or shorter, differ noticeably from your regular schedule or stop altogether for three cycles before age 45). Missed periods might also indicate other health issues. If you don't take hormone therapy, also known as hormone "replacement" therapy in this situation, you run the danger of developing a number of long-term health issues, such as heart disease, dementia, Parkinsonism, and osteoporosis if you are going through premature or early menopause. Your doctor can assist in deciding whether you are in fact going through early or premature menopause.

2. The long-term health effects of early or premature menopause must be mitigated with hormone therapy. The North American Menopause Society and other expert medical groups advise using hormone therapy at least until the natural age of menopause (age 51) unless there is a very good reason to avoid it in your individual situation. However, some of the effects of early estrogen loss, such as mood swings and sexual dysfunction, may not be fully alleviated by hormone therapy.

3. Plans for your family could be altered. If you want to start a family, you may need to think about possibilities like storing eggs or embryos. If you had intended to have children, you might need to give yourself permission to entertain a new aspiration, such as starting a family through surrogacy, adoption, or in vitro fertilization using donor eggs.

4. You can regain your sexuality. Consult your healthcare professional if you have a dry vagina or poor sexual desire. Vaginal dryness may be helped with estrogen-based hormonal therapy. In rare cases, testosterone medication may even be appropriate for women with decreased sexual desire who experience early or premature menopause. Talk to your partner as well. Higher levels of sexual satisfaction are correlated with effective communication.

5. You might need further assistance. If you are going through early or premature menopause, you may need more time and assistance to accept your diagnosis and all of its implications, including the loss of fertility and potential long-term health effects. It can be beneficial to discuss your worries with your partner, close friends, and your doctor or psychologist. The key is to comprehend what is occurring in your body and what you can do to stop it.

❖ THE REALITY OF TYPICAL MENOPAUSE MYTHS

For almost half of the population, the change from perimenopause to menopause is a totally normal aspect of life. There is still a stigma attached to it, though. This opens the door to miscommunication and unwarranted anxiety.

Discover the reality behind these typical menopause myths and learn some basic information.

Myth #1: Menopause starts late in life

The transition typically begins in midlife, but it can begin earlier or later.

You are in menopause if you haven't had a period in a year. However, perimenopause refers to the changes that occur before menopause and begin much earlier.

Menopause typically occurs between ages in the United States, but:

➢ Menopause affects 5% of women between the ages of 40 and 45.
➢ 1% of women reach menopause before the age of 40.

The average age of natural menopause, according to a 2014 review of 46 studies from 24 different nations, was 48.8 years old. The study contends that various nations, regions, and ethnic groups have varying menopause ages.

These elements could contribute to these differences:

➢ Genetic differences
➢ Social and economic standing
➢ environment
➢ Early childhood and reproductive considerations

The time of menopause may also be influenced by other lifestyle factors, such as:

➢ smoking
➢ education, employment, and wealth.
➢ Body mass index and level of physical activity (BMI)

Myth #2: Everybody has the same menopausal experience

Menopause is not a common occurrence for everyone. Not everyone experiences the same signs or intensity levels.

For women of color, perimenopause may begin earlier and last longer than it does for non-Latina white women. According to certain studies, Latina women and non-Latina black women experienced hot flashes, insomnia, and sadness more frequently, whereas non-Latina Asian women were more likely to report a decline in sex drive.

The following variables could affect how you react to menopause:

➢ Personal convictions
➢ cultural values
➢ income level
➢ discrimination
➢ general environment

Myth #3: Menopause only lasts a brief period of time

The menopause transition lasts for years for the majority of women. When the ovaries decrease estrogen and progesterone production, perimenopause begins. Each individual experiences this at a different rate.

Myth #4: Menopause is unpleasant

Menopausal symptoms are typically mild to moderate for the majority of people. When you think about certain parts of menopause, it may be wonderfully liberating—even for those who have more distressing, disruptive symptoms:

➤ Premenstrual syndrome (PMS) disappears completely.
➤ Periods, period-related products, and other items related to menstrual cycles are no longer available.
➤ You can put an end to worries about an unforeseen pregnancy or the requirement for birth control. (However, you'll still need protection from sexually transmitted infection's if you're not monogamous.)

Myth #5: Menopause destroys your sexual drive

Your sex drive doesn't disappear when you go through menopause. A fulfilling sex life is still possible. Some people may find it freeing and downright attractive to be rid of their period and birth control.

Your sex drive may be affected by lower hormone levels during perimenopause and menopause. But not everyone experiences that.

Additionally, some menopause symptoms, such as vaginal dryness, can make having sex painful or uncomfortable.

If you're not into sex, that's okay too. You are not required to stop having sex, though, if you don't want to.

Several of the following are helpful:

➢ Moisturizers for the vagina can help with dryness.

➢ Use lubricants to make sexual contact less painful.

➢ Have more intercourse to help the blood flow, which in turn helps to maintain the health of the vaginal tissues.

➢ Foreplay is essential as becoming completely aroused also causes a rise in natural wetness.

➢ Find your comfort zone by trying out new positions.

➢ Exercise your pelvic floor to build muscles and increase blood flow to the area.

➢ Avoid irritating goods like soaps with strong scents.

➢ Consult your doctor about hormone replacement therapy or prescription-strength drugs that may help make sex more bearable.

Myth #6: Hot flashes and night sweats are unavoidable symptoms

Uncomfortable menopausal vasomotor symptoms (MVS), such as hot flashes and night sweats, can be treated using a variety of methods. Your face and upper body experience a burst of heat during a hot flash. It can be highly disturbing and last for a few seconds or several minutes. Night sweats may develop as well, which can keep you from sleeping. Some individuals may endure the occasional hot flash. However, it becomes a significant issue when symptoms are severe or overly frequent.

Here are a few tactics that could be useful:

➢ Avoid triggers like alcohol, hot drinks like coffee and tea, and spicy foods.

➢ Layer your clothing to make it easier to cool off when you sense a flash approach.

➢ Drink cool water when a heat flash first appears. While you sleep, keep an iced water thermos next to your bed, and maintain a supply of ice packs in your freezer that is ready to use.

➢ Choose breathable materials for your pajamas and bedding.

Additionally, you can discuss therapy possibilities like:

➢ treatment with either estrogen or estrogen and progesterone. These could come in the form of pills, skin patches, or vaginal lotions. Non-hormonal medications used to treat insomnia, night sweats, and hot flashes

Myth #7: Menopause denotes advanced age

Menopause is a significant stage of life, but it doesn't make you seem older. Menopause might begin in your 30s if you think of your age in terms of numbers. Therefore, it is unquestionably not an old-age sign. Simply put, menopause is a new stage of life. It can be unpredictable and possibly fruitful, just like every other phase you've gone through.

COMPLICATIONS

Your risk of developing some medical disorders rises after menopause.

Examples include:

Cardiovascular disease (heart and blood vessel problems)

Your risk of developing cardiovascular disease increases when your estrogen levels drop. Therefore, it's crucial to keep a normal weight, engage in regular exercise, and consume a healthy diet. Ask your doctor for tips on how to keep your heart healthy, such as how to lower your blood pressure or cholesterol if it's too high.

Osteoporosis

This disorder makes bones weak and brittle, which increases the chance of fractures. You may experience rapid bone density loss in the first few years following menopause, which raises your risk of osteoporosis. Osteoporotic postmenopausal women are particularly prone to wrist, hip, and spine fractures.

Urinary incontinence

You may have frequent, sudden, strong urges to urinate, followed by an uncontrollable loss of urine (urge incontinence), or the loss of urine with coughing, laughing, or raising as the tissues of your vagina and urethra lose their suppleness (stress incontinence). Urinary tract infections might occur more frequently for you.

Using topical vaginal estrogen and strengthening your pelvic floor muscles with Kegel exercises may help you feel less incontinent. Menopausal vaginal and urinary tract abnormalities that might cause urine incontinence may also be successfully treated with hormone therapy.

Sexual activity

During sexual activity, vaginal dryness brought on by decreased moisture production and elasticity loss can cause discomfort and very minor bleeding. Reduced feelings may also lessen your desire for sexual action (libido).

Water-based vaginal lubricants and moisturizers may be beneficial. Many women find it helpful to use local vaginal estrogen treatment, which comes in the form of a vaginal cream, pill, or ring if a vaginal lubricant isn't sufficient.

Weight gain

Weight gain Because of a slowed metabolism, many women put on weight throughout the menopausal transition and later. To keep your weight stable, you might need to eat less and move more.

CHAPTER 2: MENOPAUSE & BOWEL CHANGES

All women eventually go through menopause, which is a natural part of life. Despite the fact that many women are relieved to be menstruation-free, menopause also brings up additional uncomfortable symptoms. Bowel changes may become more frequent in women, which can be uncomfortable and embarrassing. Even though menopausal women frequently experience gastrointestinal changes, maintaining healthy behaviors is important for controlling uncomfortable symptoms.

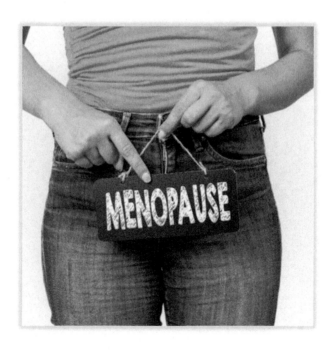

Menopause

As a woman ages, the amount of estrogen in her body decreases, and menstrual periods eventually stop. This is known as menopause. Before menopause is fully enacted, menstrual periods may be erratic for months or even years. Menopause-related hormonal changes can also result in other unwanted symptoms like dry vaginal passages, hot flashes, and thinning hair. Many women going through menopause frequently complain about their bowel changes.

Large Intestine

The large intestine, often known as the gut, has a number of uses. The leftovers proceed into the large intestine where they are transformed into the stool for disposal after food digestion and nutrient absorption in the stomach and small intestine. Vitamins and water are absorbed when waste passes through the colon before leaving the body.

Constipation

During menopause, hormones might fluctuate, which can result in constipation. Many women who have additional menopausal symptoms may eat to relieve stress, and eating poorly can also cause constipation.

Constipation may be a side effect of some drugs used to treat menopause symptoms, such as vitamin supplements and sleep aids. According to Menopause Insight, constipation is characterized by less than three stools per week, the appearance of firm stools, and straining or difficulty during bowel movements.

Gas

Some women express increased discomfort from flatulence and gas pain. Food breakdown during the digestive process results in gas. Some vegetables, like broccoli, beans, and cabbage, cause more gas than others. Some menopausal women strive to eat a healthy diet to feel better and increase their intake of fruits and vegetables every day, which might cause indigestion and discomfort. Increased gas, bloating, and flatulence during menopause are also linked to a drop in hormone production.

Prevention/Solution

Menopause bowel change symptoms can be avoided by eating a healthy diet rich in fiber, engaging in regular exercise, and drinking lots of water. Constipation can be eased and supported by eight to ten glasses of water per day. Additionally, women who experience excessive bloating may take over-the-counter drugs that reduce gas.

MIDDLE AGE BLOATING & BELLY FAT

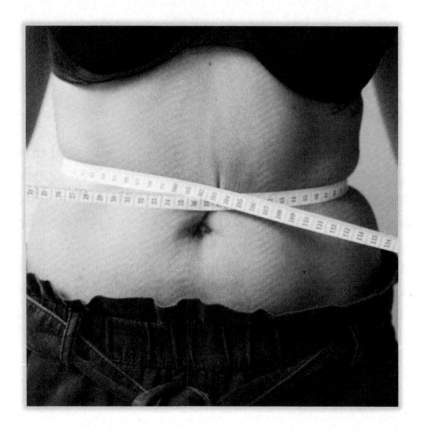

Physical discomfort and self-consciousness are brought on by middle-aged belly fat and increased bloating.

According to the National Institute on Aging, at this stage of life, both men and women are more likely to develop belly fat and lose lean tissue. The age-related slowing of your metabolism and consuming more calories than you expend lead to an increase in belly fat. Visceral fat, the fat around your organs that poses a major health concern, is a component of belly fat. Bloating and belly fat can be reduced through healthy practices.

Changes

As you age, your digestion changes. You might find that you digest meals more slowly and that you react poorly to some foods. Many individuals dislike lactose, the sugar found in milk. Your digestion may also be hampered by wheat, other grains, beans, and peanuts, or they may cause food sensitivities. Hormonal changes can cause bloating and tummy obesity in women in their middle years. Both men and women appear bloated because of water retention caused by sodium ingestion.

Bloating

Constipation, gas, irritable bowel syndrome, overeating, a tendency to swallow air when stressed, smoking, intolerance to lactose or other foods, and irritable bowel syndrome can all contribute to abdominal bloating. Bloating can occasionally be brought on by a significant medical condition. If you have any medical worries, consult your doctor. Finding the reason for the bloating is made easier by keeping a food log. Gas can be brought on by beans and cruciferous foods like broccoli and cabbage. Consuming these nutritious foods in moderation and taking a digestive enzyme supplement can help.

Belly Fat

Two types of fat are stored in your belly. The layer under the skin is known as subcutaneous fat. According to a Rush University Medical Center report, visceral fat, which builds up around your important organs and raises your risk of heart disease, stroke, and type-2 diabetes, does not pose the same serious health risks as body fat. Alcohol is another factor in belly obesity. You must cut back on calories while increasing your regular physical activity if you want to successfully lose belly fat.

Tips

Gas and bloating can be avoided by avoiding fatty foods, chewing gum, smoking, carbonated beverages, and eating more slowly to avoid swallowing air. To lessen bloating, try eating more fiber to prevent constipation and add yogurt or probiotic supplements to your diet. Exercises that combine resistance training with cardiovascular conditioning, such as circuit training with free weights, interval training, aerobic dance, and workouts, as well as vigorous movement, are effective strategies to burn fat. Weight-bearing exercises, such as resistance training, help you maintain your metabolism as you become older and keep your bones strong.

HOW TO LOSE MENOPAUSAL BELLY FAT

Menopause is a normal aspect of becoming older. Additionally, it is typical for this hormonal change to result in weight gain. But learning how to lose menopause belly fat can be helpful if your objective is to lose that weight.

According to the National Institute on Aging, menopause starts when your monthly cycle ceases (often between the ages of 45 and 55) as a result of a natural decline in female reproductive hormones, including estrogen and progesterone (NIA). Menopause is referred to as a transition since it might take up to seven years to complete.

According to the NIA, weight gain is typical during menopause as your body adjusts to a change in how it processes energy. In addition to weight gain, you might additionally suffer from the following symptoms:

➢ Hot flashes
➢ Mood changes
➢ Difficulty sleeping
➢ Headaches
➢ Sexual discomfort
➢ Reduced bone density

Here are some suggestions on how to lose menopausal belly fat if you're wondering how to regain your waistline after menopause.

❖ Eat a Balanced Diet

The methods for losing weight during menopause are largely the same as those used for other times of life. And one crucial strategy is eating a wholesome menopausal diet.

Here are some considerations to make when you create the ideal diet to reduce belly fat associated with menopause.

1. Reduce your calorie intake

Menopausal women may develop visceral fat, or belly fat, which is fat that is located inside the abdominal wall. Your internal organs are encircled by this sort of fat, which has been linked to diseases including heart disease.

Fortunately, when you start to lose weight, visceral fat is among the first fats you'll burn. A daily calorie deficit, or eating fewer calories than you burn, is one approach to achieving this.

You can lose weight at a healthy and sustainable rate of 1 to 2 pounds per week by maintaining a daily caloric deficit of 500 to 1,000 calories. Simply deduct your ideal calorie deficit from your current daily calorie intake to find out how many calories you should consume each day to lose weight.

What Are Your Daily Calorie Requirements?

The 2020–2025 Dietary Guidelines for Americans recommend that people who were assigned female at birth (AFAB) consume the following number of calories each day, depending on their level of activity:

➢ 1,600 calories if they are not active.
➢ For moderate exercise, 1,800 calories for
➢ 2,200 to 2,400 calories from exercise.

2. Get Enough Protein

You begin to lose muscle as you get older. However, consuming a lot of protein can help counteract that muscle loss. Additionally, it can support your energy levels throughout the day, including during exercise, another essential element of any weight-loss plan.

Some dependable protein sources include:

➢ Lean meats, such as poultry and turkey,
➢ Fish such as tuna and salmon
➢ Tofu and other soy products.
➢ seeds and nuts.
➢ Beans
➢ "Grains high in protein"
➢ Eggs
➢ Yogurt and cottage cheese are examples of dairy products.

The Dietary Guidelines for Americans recommend that people with AFAB who are 50 years of age or older have 5 to 6-ounce equivalents of protein daily. The amount of protein that "counts" as an ounce is known as an ounce equivalent, and examples include an egg, a tablespoon of peanut butter, a quart cup of cooked beans, and a half ounce of almonds.

3. Consume plenty of fiber

Another crucial ingredient for feeling your best and shedding pounds is fiber. It promotes healthy digestion, regulates bowel movements, and aids in blood sugar stabilization. Because fiber fills you up and keeps you from eating more than you need to, it may also encourage weight loss.

Include the following fiber-rich foods in your diet to reduce belly fat and menopause symptoms:

➢ Vegetables and fruits.
➢ seeds and nuts.
➢ Beans
➢ Whole grains like spelled and oats

4. Reduce or avoid processed foods

Processed foods with a lot of calories can make you gain weight without giving you any extra nutrition. It's important to minimize or stay away from foods like:

➢ Rough carbohydrates, such as white bread,
➢ foods like soda and sauces that have been sweetened.
➢ Fried items

➢ Bakery products

Warning

Avoid eating less than 1,200 calories per day (unless your doctor has prescribed it), as you risk missing out on important nutrients.

❖ Exercise consistently

Another essential component of how to lose menopausal abdominal fat is regular exercise. To get started, consider these tips:

1. Start a cardio program

Your daily calorie deficit may be aided by increasing your activity level, which will increase your daily caloric burn. The Physical Activity Guidelines for Americans state that people should strive to complete 150 minutes of moderate-intensity exercise (or 75 minutes of intense cardio).

A quick walk around your neighborhood qualifies as moderate-intensity exercise, so you don't have to spend hours on an elliptical or treadmill.

Other aerobic exercises consist of:

➤ Water exercise
➤ Swimming
➤ Biking
➤ Tennis
➤ Dancing
➤ Gardening and other outside chores

Tips

1. If you want to have fun and lose weight without putting too much strain on your joints, try low-impact cardio exercises like swimming or water walking.

2. Don't forget to do strength training

According to the Mayo Clinic, as you age, your muscle mass and bone density start to decrease. In addition to eating a lot of protein, strength training is an essential component in maintaining muscle and bone strength.

Two strength-training sessions per week are advised for adults by the Physical Activity Guidelines for Americans. Uncertain about where to start? By working with a fitness professional, you can create a strength-building program that is safe, effective and suited to your mobility, flexibility, balance, and objectives. You might wish to try any of the popular forms of strength training listed below:

➢ Weight lifting
➢ Circuit training
➢ Isometric exercise

CHAPTER 3: WEIGHT GAIN DURING MENOPAUSE

Although most women gain weight as they age, extra weight is not always present. Increase your activity level and consume a balanced diet to reduce menopause weight gain.

It's probable that maintaining your regular weight becomes harder as you get older. In reality, a large number of women gain weight as they enter menopause. However, the weight increase is not necessarily a certainty during menopause. You can change your situation by practicing healthy eating habits and having an active lifestyle.

What causes weight gain during menopause?

As a result of the hormonal changes brought on by menopause, you may be more likely to gain weight in your midsection than in your hips and thighs. But menopause weight gain isn't always brought on by hormonal changes alone.

Instead, weight growth is often correlated with aging, lifestyle choices, and hereditary factors.

For instance, while muscle mass typically increases with age, the fat tends to increase. If you have less muscle mass, your body uses calories more slowly (metabolism). As a result, maintaining a healthy weight may become more challenging. If you continue eating the same things you usually have and don't up your physical activity, you're likely to gain weight.

Genetic factors may also affect weight gain during menopause. If your parents or other close relatives are overweight in the middle, you probably will be as well. Menopause weight gain may also be influenced by other factors like inactivity, poor eating habits, and insufficient sleep. Lack of sleep makes people more likely to overeat and snack more frequently.

How risky is weight gain after menopause?

Putting on weight while going through menopause could be harmful to your health. Being overweight increases your risk of developing a number of ailments, including:
- ➤ Breathing issues
- ➤ Cardiovascular disease
- ➤ Diabetes type 2

Being overweight also increases your risk of developing uterine, colon, or breast cancer.

WHAT IS THE BEST WAY TO PREVENT PUTTING ON WEIGHT AFTER MENOPAUSE?

There is no secret formula for preventing or reversing menopause weight gain. Remain focused on the basics of weight management:

Increase your activity

You can lose extra weight and keep it off by engaging in physical activity such as strength training and aerobic exercise. Your body burns calories more effectively when you put on muscle, which makes it easier to maintain a healthy weight.

Most healthy individuals should engage in strong aerobic activity, such as jogging, for at least 75 minutes per week or moderate aerobic activity, such as brisk walking, for at least 150 minutes per week.

Furthermore, weight training exercises should be performed at least twice each week. You might need to exercise more if you want to shed weight or achieve specific fitness goals.

Eat less

You may require 200 fewer calories per day in your fifties than you needed in your thirties and forties to maintain your weight, let alone shed more pounds.

Be mindful of your eating and drinking habits if you want to cut calories without sacrificing nutrition. Increase your consumption of fruits, vegetables, and whole grains, especially those that are less processed and higher in fiber.

A plant-based diet is often better for you than other options. Good options include fish, soy, almonds, legumes, and low-fat dairy products. Limit your consumption of meat, especially chicken and red meat. Use oils like olive or vegetable oil in place of butter, stick margarine, and shortening.

Examine your sweet routine

In the typical American diet, added sugars make up roughly 300 calories per day. Most of these calories—about half of them—come from sugar-sweetened liquids such as flavored beverages, juices, energy drinks, flavored waters, and sweetened coffee and tea.

Cookies, pies, cakes, doughnuts, ice cream, and candy are other foods that increase dietary sugar intake.

Limit alcohol

Drinking alcohol increases your risk of gaining weight since it adds extra calories to your diet.

Ask for help

Be in the company of loved ones and friends who will support your attempts to adopt a healthy diet and improve your level of physical activity. Even better, form a team and alter your lifestyle as a whole.

A lasting change in food and exercise routines is necessary for weight loss success at any stage of life. Make a commitment to a healthier you by adopting new habits.

IN MIDLIFE, YOUR METABOLISM ACCELERATES.

You can thank middle age for the tighter fit of your clothing these days. Our metabolism slows as we get older. Learn how to increase your metabolism and shed extra weight.

Have you noticed that, ahem, your clothing is feeling a little snug lately? You continue to eat the same way you always did and go for daily walks. Why then, should you be putting on weight?

The middle age

Our metabolism, the mechanism by which we burn calories to maintain a healthy weight, slows down as we get older. All of a sudden, the additional bowl of ice cream you regularly have before bed starts to appear on your hips and thighs.

Not to worry; all you need to do is raise the thermostat a little while reducing your fuel consumption. This is especially crucial in the years immediately following menopause when studies show that women tend to put on weight a little bit more quickly than they do later in life or before menopause. Why?

Though the exact link between menopause and these changes in body composition (less muscle and more fat) and fat distribution within the body is unclear to researchers, Since muscle cells consume more fuel than fat cells do, having less muscle will result in a slower metabolism.

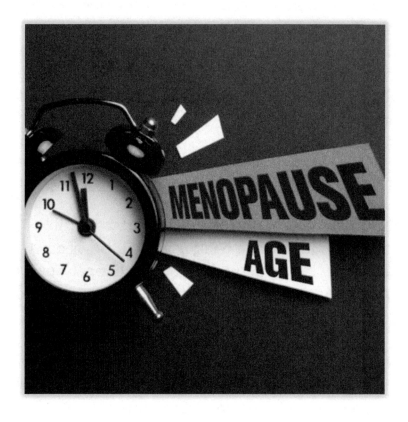

Regarding the distribution of fat, it is more likely that after menopause your abdomen will develop fat than your thighs and hips. This harmful type of fat in your abdomen, known as "visceral" fat, raises your risk of diabetes and heart disease. Women who receive estrogen therapy after menopause tend to have less abdominal fat; therefore, it appears that estrogen is somehow connected to this alteration.

To control your fat distribution, however, we do not advise using estrogen therapy. Although taking estrogen therapy has many benefits, reducing belly fat is not one of them.

Instead, sticking to those two tried-and-true methods of food and exercise, especially exercise, is your best choice. Physical activity, not age or food, was found to have the biggest impact when total body fat and abdominal body fat measurements were compared in middle-aged female twins.

Who, however, have time for exercise when they are chasing after their children around town, juggling a demanding job, discovering new opportunities in life, preserving their relationships, taking care of their elderly parents, etc. It should come as no surprise that just 50% of women between the ages of 50 and 64 report engaging in any regular physical activity, and only 14% report engaging in any vigorous exercise (such as an aerobics class or jogging).

What makes the physical activity so crucial? Because physical activity increases calorie burn, not just during exercise but also later, whereas dieting just impacts the number of calories you consume. Your metabolism is rising along with your muscular mass. You burn more calories per hour, and the faster your metabolism is. You'll lose weight the more calories you burn per hour (or at least not gain).

There are many benefits to engaging in consistent physical activity, even if you're content with your weight. Here are only a few instances:

➢ prolonging life. A significant study found that exercise decreased postmenopausal women risk factors for all types of mortality.

➢ establishing a regular workout routine. According to studies, whether you'll continue to exercise after menopause depends heavily on how you feel throughout the perimenopausal stage, which lasts from your mid-30s to your 40s.

➢ Boosting "good" cholesterol levels while lowering blood pressure and "bad" cholesterol levels.

➢ slowing your resting heart rate, allowing your heart to beat more efficiently

➢ It lowers your risk of developing a divers illness, kidney stones, colon cancer, and gallstone surgery.

➢ Breast cancer risk reduction; bone density enhancement and osteoporosis prevention

➢ promoting deeper, more restful sleep.

➢ enhancing your emotional condition while reducing depression or just making you feel better overall.

➢ help you with stress management.

Nobody is encouraging you to go on a five-mile run. Simply add some movement to your daily activities. For instance, did you know that walking for around 30 minutes a day at a rate that leaves you gasping for air can reduce your risk of heart disease by more than a third?

What about:

➢ Surrender to the power tools. Cancel the lawn service and put the riding mower and leaf blower back in the garage. Do your own yard work and enter the garden. Gardening is one of the best ways to keep your bones strong after menopause.

➢ Walking first, then driving. When doing your weekly shopping, park at the far end of the parking lot, go inside restaurants to grab your food, then make one more lap around the grocery store.

➢ Collaborating with another female. If you know your neighbor is waiting for you, you're considerably more inclined to get up at 6 in the morning on a chilly morning.

➢ You can create a gym in your home. Pace around your home while you're on the phone, carry your own heavy packages into the house twice, and run up and down the stairs for 20 minutes each day while using gallon milk jugs as weights.

➢ Divide up your workouts into shorter intervals. You can't find 30 minutes to go for that two-mile walk. Take the dog for a 10-minute stroll three times per day. The advantages are the same for you.

One caution: aim for an hour or two of resistance training per week, such as weightlifting, Pilates or yoga, or even calisthenics (knee bends, lunges, pull-ups, push-ups, etc.). These exercises are crucial for enhancing and maintaining muscular tone as well as for calorie burning. As we age, maintaining our balance and remaining solid on our feet depends on muscle tone.

Make a chart and note the days you exercise for at least 30 minutes. It will take around two to three weeks before it becomes routine, just like with any new habit. Then it will become such a routine part of your life that you'll feel strange on the days you forget to do it, just like fastening your seat belt when you get into your car or brushing your teeth before bed.

What Is the Relationship Between Estrogen and Weight Gain?

Weight gain is common among postmenopausal women, especially in the abdomen. Part of the problem is estrogen loss, but there are techniques to combat it. What part does estrogen play in weight growth, you might be wondering? You have every right to ask that, too. You know you can't win, right? High estrogen levels are problematic. When it's high, it contributes to symptoms that you're probably already familiar with, such as heavy bleeding, irregular periods, PMS, endometriosis, fibroids, lethargy, mood swings, and occasionally breast or ovarian cancer. It also has an impact on us when it is low. Missed or irregular periods, infertility, and mood swings are largely the same. Anything else, um? I'm sure there are more. Yes, there are other issues related to menopause. One is weak bones. heat blasts for another Additionally, there is a rise in urinary tract infections and—let's face it—the big one—weight gain. I'm sorry, but you were already aware of that. For many menopausal women, low estrogen levels can cause weight gain. What actually occurs, then? Women frequently become aware of weight gain or find it more challenging to shed weight. During menopause, estradiol, an estrogen sub-type, declines. Your body weight and metabolism are both regulated by estradiol. Hence the problems with weight. Why does that weight choose to accumulate in the midsection as opposed to the hips and thighs? I'm no longer a "pear," I'm an "apple." Despite the need for greater study, some studies have revealed that "perimenopause, independent of age, is related to increased fat in the abdomen as well as decreased lean body mass." This kind of fat seems to like to migrate there. Break it to me, please. Why is being an apple more perilous than being a pear? It's because there's more going on than meets the eye. There is more to belly fat than just the extra padding you can see beneath your skin (known as subcutaneous fat). It is also visceral fat, which is the fat that surrounds your internal organs deep inside your belly and is hidden from view. Visceral fat is associated with a number of potentially fatal health issues, including heart disease, type 2 diabetes, high blood pressure, high cholesterol, and an even higher risk of dying before one's time (regardless of your overall weight).

What are the opinions of the experts?

Others point to other midlife factors that occur around the same time as menopause, such as the fact that women become less active and more sedentary (many midlife women, including this one, beg to differ), as well as a natural slowing of metabolism, in place of the low estrogen that some blame for weight gain. It seems inevitable that decreased estrogen would lead to weight gain.

Definitely not. There is compelling evidence that a combination of physical activity, a decent, healthy diet, and prudent portion control can significantly reduce weight gain that occurs throughout this stage of life. It may also be necessary to exercise more frequently than usual; nevertheless, this will be beneficial. Make sure to include strength training in your exercise routine because it increases the muscular mass that we also lose as we age while also helping to promote metabolism. Discover how to defend yourself through exercise.

Additionally, as sitting has been related to higher levels of belly fat, standing up whenever possible will be in your best interest. Move around more, stand up more, and sit down less. (A standing desk is ideal for folks who work while sitting; pacing while on the phone is also great.)

Oh, and make an effort to get a restful night's sleep. The chemicals leptin and ghrelin, which control your hunger and appetite, are activated by sleep deprivation.

Why Sleep Is So Important for Losing Weight

Although each diet or weight-loss program has its own unique approach to the process, the fundamentals always involve reducing calories while stepping up exercise. However, most strategies overlook one crucial element: your sleep.
Sleep is necessary for a healthy body, though, and it has an impact on your hormones, digestion, how fat is stored, and even your capacity for decision-making, all of which can affect how much weight you weigh.

Here's what you should know about how sleep (or lack thereof) may be hurting your weight-loss objectives if you're strictly adhering to your food plan and working out frequently but not making time for decent slumber.

1. Inadequate sleep disrupts hormonal balance

The hormones leptin and ghrelin are produced by your body depending on how much sleep you get.

Your body produces the hormone leptin to make you feel more full. Leptin controls how much you eat and how much energy you use, which aids in keeping your weight stable. However, limiting sleep might cause the body to produce less leptin. Your hunger increases as a result, which may lead you to overeat. Because of this, a late night may cause you to feel less content after lunch and turn more frequently to the snack drawer.

Your ghrelin levels increase while your leptin levels decrease when you are sleep deprived. Ghrelin is a hormone that makes you feel more hungry and makes you seek and eat more calorie-dense foods in an effort to make up for your lack of energy.

Cortisol, a hormone linked to stress, can build up in the body more as a result of sleep deprivation. Chronically high cortisol levels may have a harmful impact on your body's metabolism in addition to making you feel more hungry.

2. Shut-Eye Deficit Affects How Your Body Stores and Burns Fat

Restricted sleep can boost cortisol, which can change where your body stores fat. You tend to store extra belly fat when you are sleep deprived. This visceral adipose tissue, often known as "VAT," or abdominal fat, releases inflammatory chemicals, which raise cortisol levels. Even after just a few days, sleep deprivation can alter how your body accumulates fat from food. According to blood sample comparisons, following a meal, participants who had limited sleep maintained less fat in their bloodstream. This indicates that when sleep-deprived, the body accumulates or stores fat more quickly.

A tiny study from October 2010 that was published in the Annals of Internal Medicine found that getting less sleep can also lessen the advantages of diet and exercise. In a sleep-deprived state, calorie restriction causes your body to lose more lean muscle mass than fat. This ultimately reduces the effectiveness of your diet because muscle burns more calories than fat, even when at rest.

3. Your Circadian Rhythm Is Important for Gut Health

In the same way that hormones can influence how much you weigh, your stomach can also prevent you from losing weight. According to Dr. Li, your gut microbiome, which consists of billions of bacteria, viruses, yeast, and fungi, is crucial for digestion and the processing of food, medications, hormones, and brain chemicals. As a result, the population of helpful bacteria is crucial for maintaining weight.

People who are active at night may have poor gut health. Your circadian rhythm, your body's internal clock that controls your sleep, is impacted by sleep deprivation, which can harm your stomach.

There is a cyclical relationship between sleep deprivation and gut health. Sleep deprivation, even for brief periods, might change the bacteria in your stomach. This causes your body's inflammatory response to rise, which may result in further sleep loss.

4. The less sleep you get, the less willpower you have.

Sleep may change the type of food you crave in addition to your emotions of hunger and fullness. According to a March 2016 study published in Sleep, sleep deprivation activates areas of the brain linked to motivation and reward, which can boost food cravings, especially for unhealthy meals.

The prefrontal cortex of the brain, which is in charge of impulse control and aids in decision-making, is also badly impacted by sleep deprivation. Therefore, lack of sleep might affect both your ability to resist indulging in unhealthy meals as well as your desire for them. In studies examining the relationship between acute sleep deprivation and food preferences, those with less sleep favored high-calorie junk meals more. It is obvious that, when our bodies are worn out, we would seek "easy energy." Foods that provide "easy energy" can also be calming. Comfort foods appear to reduce stress-related symptoms when cortisol levels rise (such as when you get little sleep), which may lead you to seek more unhealthy meals.

HOW TO SLEEP BETTER

We're all occasionally guilty of staying up to watch one more episode of our favorite show or checking our email before going to bed. But breaking some poor habits and making the most of your nighttime routine will help you get a better night's sleep and prepare you for weight loss success. Give yourself ample time to unwind because your body needs to have time to transition to night mode. The National Sleep Foundation suggests creating a soothing evening routine (such as stretching or journaling) and avoiding bright light in the hours before you go to bed. Set your bedroom's temperature between 60 and 67 degrees, and abstain from alcohol and nicotine throughout the evening. Consider consulting your doctor or a sleep specialist if you continue to have trouble sleeping or experience insomnia. Some people find that maintaining a sleep journal can assist in highlighting any problematic sleeping patterns they may be engaging in unknowingly.

Words of Encouragement

If you're a woman over 50 who wants to lose weight, you could feel discouraged, frazzled, or even shocked. That's all normal; it can be difficult to lose weight during and after menopause! However, losing weight after the age of 50 is 100% possible with a little effort and knowledge of health beyond looks.

1. Recognize the changes in your body.

Nodding to puberty and noting that we all went through changes then, too, she continues, "While you should do everything you can to safeguard your health and feel your best, instead of entirely opposing the shift, recognize that these changes are a natural part of aging." She advises, "Include your blessings and count aging as one of them. Avoid fad diets; eat a little less and move around a little more, and incorporate weight training into your exercises to prevent the loss of lean body mass." in the interim.

2. There is still time

It's never too late to discover or cultivate your healthiest self, and as you age, it's crucial to avoid becoming sedentary.

As you get older, keep active since there's still time to improve your health. Do it for yourself and your family; never give up on your health. You deserve it!

3. Ignore the Scale

According to Jeffcoat, a physical therapist, she doesn't usually work with women directly on weight-loss goals and instead informs them that as they increase muscle, they may in fact gain a little weight while dropping a dress or pant size.

CHAPTER 4: THE NO-NONSENSE MENOPAUSAL WEIGHT LOSS GUIDE FOR WOMEN

Exercise on a regular basis is essential for menopausal women. Consider the advantages exercise can provide for you. Menopause marks a significant turning point in women's lives. Use it as a prompt to remember to look after yourself. Start by taking into account these menopause fitness suggestions.

Why is exercise crucial during menopause?

Exercise has numerous advantages both during and after menopause, including:

➤ Preventing weight gain. Around menopause, women frequently experience muscle loss and abdominal fat gain. Exercise on a regular basis can help stop weight gain.

➤ Cancer prevention. Exercise can help you reduce extra weight or maintain a healthy weight, which may provide protection from many types of cancer, including breast, colon, and endometrial cancer. This is true both during and after menopause.

➢ Build up your bones. After menopause, exercise helps reduce bone loss, reducing the risk of fractures and osteoporosis. lowering the likelihood of contracting more illnesses. Putting on weight while going through menopause could be harmful to your health.

➢ Type 2 diabetes and heart disease are both made more likely by excess weight. Exercise on a regular basis can reduce these hazards. It will make you feel better. Adults who are physically active are less likely to have depression or cognitive decline.

➢ Consistent exercise can improve your well-being, lessen stress, and support you in maintaining a healthy weight.

What are the best physical activities to try?

The Department of Health and Human Services recommends moderate aerobic exercise for at least 150 minutes a week or intense aerobic exercise for at least 75 minutes a week for the majority of healthy women.

Additionally, doing weight training activities at least twice a week is encouraged. Spread out your workouts throughout the week if you'd like.

Consider the advantages of your available workout options:

Aerobic exercise

By engaging in aerobic activity, you can maintain a healthy weight and lose extra weight. Try cycling, swimming, water aerobics, jogging, or brisk walking. Beginners should start with 10 minutes per day and then progressively increase the duration and intensity.

Strengthening exercises

Strength exercising on a regular basis can help you lose body fat, build stronger muscles, and burn calories more effectively. Try using weightlifting equipment, hand weights, or resistance tubing. Select a weight or resistance level that will cause your muscles to ache after approximately 12 repetitions. As you get stronger, gradually raise the weight or resistance.

Stretching

Flexibility can be increased through stretching. After each workout, set aside some time to stretch your muscles while they are still warm and pliable.

Stability and equilibrium

Exercises that increase balance increase stability and can help prevent falls. Try some easy exercises, like brushing your teeth while standing on one leg. Taijiquan and other similar exercises are also beneficial.

How do you maintain motivation?

Set attainable, reasonable objectives. For instance, instead of promising to work out more, resolve to go for a daily 30-minute walk after dinner. As you improve your level of fitness, you should frequently revise your goals. Working together with someone, such as a partner, friend, or neighbor, can also have a positive impact. Keep in mind that you don't need to visit a gym to work out. Numerous pursuits, including dance and gardening, might help enhance your health. Take the necessary time to safely warm up and cool down, whatever you decide.

EXERCISE PLAN

The overall objective, which is in line with the Physical Exercise Guidelines for Americans, is 2.5 hours of physical activity each week. That equals 30 minutes every day, five days per week.

For menopausal women over 50, the best fitness regimen will combine aerobic exercise, strength training, and balance training. The suggested weekly plan is shown below:

➢ Four times a week, aerobic exercise such as walking, running, or dancing, with a day of relaxation in between.

➢ Weight-bearing and resistance exercise three times a week, with at least one day off in between.

➢ A 10 to 15-minute stretching program at least six days a week, alternated with strength and aerobic exercises, to create a six-to-seven-day routine.

It is advised to follow a well-rounded exercise program that includes both cardio and strength training, as well as rest days and outdoor activity.

Monday: 45 minutes of cardio or aerobic activity.
Tuesday: a 30-minute resistance-training session
Wednesday: Active recovery day or rest day
Friday: a 60-minute trek or walk outside
Thursday: a 30-minute workout (including resistance training).
Saturday: 45 minutes of cardio or aerobic exercise
Sunday: is a day of rest or active recuperation.

Add Brief Movement to Your Day

You can add modest quantities of movement throughout the day to increase your overall calorie expenditure, which will aid in long-term weight loss, in addition to a scheduled workout or substantial amount of physical activity, like a 3-mile walk. You can burn more calories every day by simply moving around or fidgeting.

Consider these entertaining suggestions:

➢ Before you sit down, perform 15 to 20 squats in front of your couch as a quick way to include daily strengthening. It won't take long at all!

➢ Try performing forward and side lunges while holding onto the wall for balance as you go down the length of your hallway. Lunges in the hallway work on both balance and strength objectives.

A few inventive exercises, too:

➤ If you often employ a cleaner, think about doing it yourself: You'll burn more calories during the week and might even feel more content as a result.

➤ Challenge yourself to stroll somewhere new or enjoyable when you take a break from work: Visit your preferred retailer, take a stroll around your office building, or locate a new park. (Even if you're just walking around the mall, every step counts!)

Other suggestions for fitting brief exercise sessions into your day are as follows:

➤ Instead of going up the stairs, lunge; this is a terrific technique to develop single-leg strength.

➤ As you carry your grocery bags inside, exercise your biceps.

➤ Stretch your shoulders or rotate your spine while sitting at your workstation.

THE BEST DIET FOR MENOPAUSAL WOMEN OVER-50 TO LOSE WEIGHT

It's crucial to keep in mind that nutrition for menopausal women over 50 is very individualized, much like fitness. Even if your sister, closest friend, or coworker is roughly the same age as you, you may (and definitely do) have different vitamin needs. Working with a healthcare expert or dietitian who can assist you in creating a dietary plan that satisfies all of your objectives is always recommended. But for now, consider this advice on how to slim down as a woman over 50.

Why Do Nutritional Requirements Differ After Age 50

Women nutritional requirements change as they age, particularly after menopause. For instance, she notes that the recommended daily intake (RDA) for iron decreases from 18 milligrams to 8 milligrams per day for women who have achieved menopause because they no longer shed blood via menstruation.

Additional nutritional requirements following the menopause include:

➢ Because there is no longer a necessity to prevent fetal neural tube abnormalities (during pregnancy), folic acid consumption does not have to be as high.

➢ The RDA for calcium has been raised to 1,200 milligrams per day due to rising concern over bone health (up from 1,000 milligrams per day).

Women over 50 should concentrate on consuming healthy fats, lean protein, low-fat dairy or dairy substitutes, lots of fruits and vegetables, and healthy fats because the risk of cardiovascular disease, diabetes, and weight gain increases after menopause.

By ensuring that your bones and joints are healthy, your energy levels are high, your mood is positive, and you feel overall healthy and energetic, meeting these nutrient targets each day helps your body function at its best and can aid in weight loss.

DIET FOR WEIGHT LOSS AFTER MENOPAUSE

Menopausal and post-menopausal individuals can adopt a few simple dietary adjustments that may aid in weight loss. What are two simple methods for weight loss? Consume protein with each meal, and steer clear of processed foods.

According to some studies, 25 to 30 grams of protein are required at each meal to best promote muscle-protein synthesis.

Consider the following examples to picture 25 to 30 grams of protein:

➤ 4 ounces of animal protein (think: chicken).
➤ Cottage cheese, 1 cup
➤ 1 scoop of whey protein.

Limit or avoid highly processed foods, especially those with added sugars, to address changes in glucose metabolism, or how your body processes sugar. Examples of highly processed foods include soda, candies, and snack foods like chips. When foods or beverages are processed or prepared, sugars and syrups are added as added sugars.

In contrast to naturally occurring sugars like those in fruit or milk, these foods provide empty calories with no nutritional value. According to the 2015–2020 Dietary Guidelines for Americans, less than 10% of your daily calories should come from added sugar.

Where Do Supplements Fit In?

Consult your doctor about supplements if you are post-menopausal or approaching menopause. Given the possibility of nutritional toxicity, supplementation should be extremely targeted (consuming too much of a certain nutrient).

For instance, too much calcium can increase a person's risk of having a heart attack, and too much vitamin D can damage a person's kidneys.

As with other populations, a person's first line of defense should be making an effort to ingest nutrients through food and drink, with supplements filling in any gaps. "

The supplement sector is not strictly regulated or monitored, which increases the danger of choosing the wrong product. Manufacturers are in charge of labeling their own products, which may lead to low-quality or incorrectly labeled supplements.

These might do nothing at all and thus be a waste of money, or they might do more harm than good. You can get assistance from a licensed dietician or doctor in selecting high-quality goods for your individual requirements.

Why a calorie deficit is important

A woman's resting energy expenditure, or the number of calories she burns while at rest, is thought to decrease during and after menopause.

Although it may be tempting to follow an extremely low-calorie diet in an effort to lose weight rapidly, doing so can occasionally make it more difficult.

According to research, cutting calories too low levels results in muscle loss and a subsequent slowdown in metabolic rate.

Consequently, even while very-low-calorie diets may cause temporary weight loss, their effects on muscle mass and metabolic rate will make it difficult to maintain the loss of weight.

Additionally, a lack of calories and a decline in muscle mass can cause bone loss. This could make you more vulnerable to osteoporosis.

Maintaining a long-term healthy lifestyle will help you maintain your metabolic rate and reduce the amount of muscle mass you lose as you age.

DIETARY GUIDELINES FOR THE MENOPAUSE

The following list of four wholesome diets has been demonstrated to aid in weight loss both during and after the menopausal transition.

The low-carb diet

Numerous studies have demonstrated the effectiveness of low-carb diets for both weight loss and belly fat reduction. Several low-carb studies have included perimenopausal and postmenopausal women, but just a few of these studies have focused solely on this group.

In one of these studies, postmenopausal women who followed a low-carbohydrate diet lost 21.8 pounds (9.9 kilograms), 27.5% of their body fat, and 3.5 inches (8.9 centimeters) from their waistlines in just six months. Additionally, consuming moderate amounts of carbohydrates can still result in weight loss.

In another study, a paleo diet with about 30% of calories coming from carbohydrates led to a higher 2-year reduction in weight and abdominal fat than a low-fat diet. 55–60% of the calories in the low-fat diet came from carbohydrates.

The Mediterranean diet

Studies suggest that the Mediterranean diet may also aid in weight loss, even though it is best known for enhancing health and lowering the risk of heart disease.

Similar to studies on low-carb diets, most studies on the Mediterranean diet have included both men and women rather than just perimenopausal or postmenopausal women.

In a study of people 55 years and older, men and women who followed a Mediterranean diet significantly reduced their belly fat. Olive oil or nuts were added to their meals as supplements.

A vegetarian or vegan diet

Diets that are vegan and vegetarian have also demonstrated weight loss potential.

An allocated group in earlier studies of postmenopausal women experienced significant weight loss and improvements in health. According to a 2018 study, perimenopausal vegans had fewer severe physical symptoms and vasomotor symptoms (like hot flashes) than omnivores.

However, it has also been demonstrated that a more adaptable vegetarian strategy that incorporates dairy and eggs is effective in older women.

Diet tips that work

Here are a few other suggestions for weight loss at any age or throughout menopause.

➤ Consume a lot of protein. Protein keeps you feeling full and satisfied, boosts your metabolism, and prevents muscle loss while you're trying to lose weight.

➤ Increase your dairy intake. According to research, dairy products can aid in fat loss while maintaining muscle mass.

➤ Consume soluble fiber-rich foods. Foods high in fiber, such as flax-seed, broccoli, avocados, and Brussels sprouts, can help improve insulin sensitivity, decrease hunger, and aid in weight loss.

➤ Drink green tea. Green tea contains caffeine and epigallocatechin gallate. They might promote fat loss.

➤ Make mindful eating a habit. You might eat less as a result of mindful eating potential to lower stress levels and enhance your relationship with food.

LIFESTYLE MODIFICATIONS THAT ENCOURAGE WEIGHT LOSS DURING MENOPAUSE

Here are some suggestions for raising your quality of life and facilitating weight loss during menopause.

Get a good night's sleep

Due to hot flashes, night sweats, stress, and other physical symptoms of estrogen depletion, many menopausal women have problems falling asleep.

However, achieving and maintaining a moderate weight requires getting enough good-quality sleep.
Inadequate sleep, higher ghrelin (the "hunger hormone") levels, and lower leptin levels are all more prevalent among overweight people.

Explore psychotherapy

Women who are suffering from symptoms of low estrogen may benefit from cognitive behavioral therapy (CBT), a type of psychotherapy that has been demonstrated to aid with insomnia.
A 2019 study found that compared to women who underwent sleep hygiene instruction or sleep restriction therapy, postmenopausal women who received CBT for their insomnia had a larger gain in sleep duration over 6 months.

CBT includes sleep restriction therapy. The goal of sleep restriction therapy is to shorten the amount of time you are awake in bed or otherwise not sleeping.

Try acupuncture

Also beneficial might be acupuncture.

In one study, over the course of six months, the frequency of hot flashes decreased by 36.7%. An analysis of numerous studies discovered that acupuncture may raise estrogen levels, which can aid in symptom relief and improve sleep.

Find a way to relieve stress

Management of stress is also essential throughout the menopausal transition.

Stress raises cortisol levels, which are linked to more belly fat in addition to raising the risk of heart disease. Numerous studies have revealed that yoga can ease menopausal symptoms and lower stress in female participants.

When to visit the doctor

Although many women do, not all of them gain weight as a result of menopause. It might be really advantageous to take charge of your weight.

If you haven't yet entered menopause, you may want to start altering your lifestyle right now to minimize its consequences. It's still not too late if you're in the middle of menopause; just make little adjustments at a time until they become a habit.

As soon as you begin exercising more and improving your diet, you'll undoubtedly see a difference. Even if maintaining a weight loss plan is difficult, doing so will improve how you look and feel.

Even though they make significant lifestyle changes, some women still struggle with weight concerns after menopause. You should consult a physician if you are gaining weight while reducing your calorie intake and engaging in regular exercise because this could be an indication of an underlying medical condition.

CHAPTER 5: OSTEOPOROSIS

Bones weakened and brittle due to osteoporosis are so easily broken by even slight stresses like coughing or bending over. Hip, wrist, and spine fractures are the most frequent ones brought on by osteoporosis.

Since bone is a living tissue, it deteriorates and is replenished continuously. When there is insufficient bone formation to replace the bone that is being lost, osteoporosis develops.

All races are susceptible to osteoporosis. Women of color and Asian women are more at risk, especially older women who have gone through menopause. Medication, a good diet, and weight-bearing exercise can all help to strengthen existing brittle bones or halt bone loss.

Symptoms

There are frequently no signs in the early stages of bone loss. However, after osteoporosis has weakened your bones, you may experience a variety of indications and symptoms, such as back discomfort brought on by a shattered or collapsing vertebra.

➢ Height loss over time
➢ A hunched position

➢ A bone that fractures substantially more quickly than anticipated.

When to visit the doctor

You might want to talk to your doctor about osteoporosis if you went through early menopause, used corticosteroids for a long time, or if either one or both of your parents had hip fractures.

Causes

New bone is created and old bone is broken down as your bones are constantly being renewed. Your bone mass increases when you're young because your body produces new bone more quickly than it destroys old bone. The majority of people reach their peak bone mass by age 30 after this process slows down in their early 20s. Bone mass decreases more quickly with aging than it is gained.

Your bone mass from your youth has a bearing on how likely you are to acquire osteoporosis. Peak bone mass differs by ethnicity and is partially inherited. The more bone you have "in the bank" and the higher your peak bone mass, the less likely it is that you will get osteoporosis as you get older.

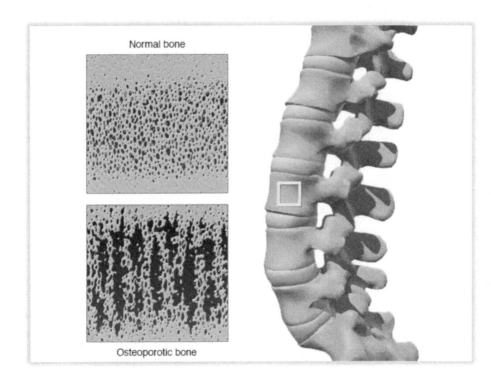

Normal bone

Osteoporotic bone

Risk factors

Your age, race, lifestyle choices, existing medical issues, and course of treatment are just a few of the variables that can make you more likely to develop osteoporosis.

Unchangeable risks

You have no control over a few osteoporosis risk factors, such as:

➢ Your sexuality.Women experience osteoporosis much more frequently than males do.

➢ Age. As you become older, your osteoporosis risk rises.

➢ Race. Your risk of osteoporosis is highest if you are white or have Asian ancestry.

➢ History of the family. You are more vulnerable if one of your parents or siblings has osteoporosis, especially if they have shattered a hip.

➢ Body frame size. Petite men and women are especially susceptible to this illness because they may have less bone mass to draw from as they age.

Hormone levels

People with excess or insufficient levels of particular hormones in their bodies are more likely to develop osteoporosis. Examples comprise:

➢ **Sexual hormones.** Bone deteriorates when sex hormone levels are low. One of the biggest risk factors for osteoporosis in women is the drop in estrogen levels throughout menopause. Treatments for breast cancer that lower estrogen levels in women and prostate cancer treatments that lower testosterone levels in men are likely to hasten bone loss.

➢ **Thyroid problems.** Bone loss can result from an excess of thyroid hormone. If your thyroid is overactive or you take too much thyroid hormone medicine to treat an under-active thyroid, this may happen.

➢ **Various glands.** Also linked to osteoporosis are hyperactive parathyroid and adrenal glands.

Dietary elements

It is more likely for someone to get osteoporosis if they have:

➢ low calcium consumption. A chronic calcium shortage leads to osteoporosis. Reduced bone density, early bone loss, and fracture risk are all increased by low calcium intake.

➢ Eating disorders. When a person significantly restricts their food intake and is underweight, their bones weaken. This applies to both men and women.

➢ Gastrointestinal surgery. The amount of surface area accessible to absorb nutrients, including calcium, is limited when your stomach is surgically reduced in size or a portion of your intestine is removed. These operations include gastrointestinal problems and weight loss.

Steroids in addition to other drugs

The process of repairing bones is hampered by the long-term usage of oral or injectable corticosteroid drugs like prednisone and cortisone. Another connection between osteoporosis and drugs used to treat or prevent it:

➢ Seizures
➢ Stomach reflux
➢ Cancer
➢ Transplant failure

Medical issues

Osteoporosis is more common in people with a number of medical conditions, including:

- Celiac illness
- Inflammation of the bowels
- liver or kidney disease.
- Cancer
- Numerous myeloma
- Inflammatory arthritis

Choices in lifestyle

Your risk of osteoporosis may rise as a result of some unhealthy behaviors. Examples comprise:

- sedentary way of life. Osteoporosis is more common in people who spend a lot of time sitting down than it is in those who are more active. Any weight-bearing exercise, as well as posture and balance-improving activities, will be beneficial to your bones, but walking, running, leaping, dancing, and weightlifting seem to be especially beneficial.

- Excessive alcoholic beverage use.Regularly consuming more than two alcoholic beverages every day raises your risk of developing osteoporosis.

- Use of tobacco. Although the precise effect that tobacco has on osteoporosis is unclear, it has been established that smoking weakens bones.

Complications

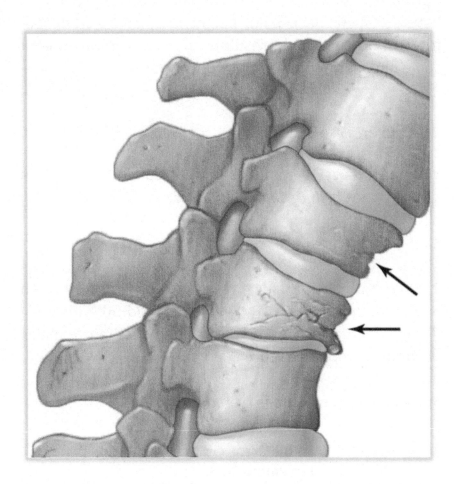

Bone fractures, particularly those that occur in the spine or hip, are the most important adverse effects of osteoporosis. Hip fractures caused by falls can cause disability and even increase the chance of death during the first year of the injury.

Vertebral fractures can occasionally occur even if you haven't fallen. Back pain, height loss, and a hunched-forward posture might result from the vertebrae in your spine becoming so weak that they collapse.

❖ Prevention

You must eat well and exercise frequently to retain strong bones for the rest of your life.

1. Calcium

1,000 mg of calcium per day is necessary for both men and women between the ages of 18 and 50. This daily dosage increases to 1,200 milligrams when females become 50 and males turn 70.

Suitable calcium sources include:

➢ Low-fat dairy items
➢ Leafy dark green vegetables
➢ Salmon or sardines in cans.
➢ Products made from soy, like tofu,
➢ Cereals supplemented with calcium and orange juice

Consider taking calcium supplements if your diet doesn't provide you with adequate calcium. However, an overabundance of calcium has been linked to kidney stones. Some experts claim that extra calcium, especially from supplements, can increase the risk of heart disease even if the exact explanation of this is still unknown.

For individuals over 50, it is advised to limit daily calcium intake to no more than 2,000 mg from supplements and diet combined.

2. Vitamin D

The body's capacity to absorb calcium is increased by vitamin D, in addition to other ways that it benefits bone health. Sunlight is one way that people can get some of their vitamin D, but if you live in a high latitude, are restricted to your home, constantly use sunscreen, or avoid the sun to lower your risk of skin cancer, this may not be the ideal source for you. Vitamin D can be obtained through the food in the forms of cod liver oil, salmon, and trout. There are numerous milk and cereal varieties that have vitamin D added to them.

Most individuals need 600 international units (IU) or more of vitamin D each day. When you reach 70 years old, you should be taking 800 IU daily.

Those without access to other vitamin D sources, especially those with little sun exposure, may require a supplement. Between 600 and 800 IU of vitamin D are found in the majority of multivitamin formulations. For the majority of people, 4,000 IU of vitamin D daily is safe.

3. Exercise

By exercising, you can slow bone loss and strengthen your bones. Exercise is good for your bones no matter when you start, but you'll gain the most if you start regularly when you're young and keep doing it as you age.

Combine exercises that require weight-bearing, balance, and strength. Your bones, arms, and upper spine will benefit from strength training. The bones in your legs, hips and lower spine are mostly influenced by weight-bearing workouts including walking, running, sprinting, stair climbing, skipping rope, and impact-producing sports. Especially as you age, tai chi and other balance activities can help lower your chance of falling.

EXERCISE AND OSTEOPOROSIS

You could be under the impression that activity will cause a fracture if you have osteoporosis. However, utilizing your muscles actually helps to safeguard your bones.

For elderly women, osteoporosis is a major source of impairment. Osteoporosis, a condition that weakens the bones, frequently causes hip and spine fractures, which can seriously limit your mobility and independence.

How can you lower your risk of suffering these potentially fatal injuries? Exercise has benefits.

While some forms of exercise are intended to improve your balance, which can help prevent falls, other forms are designed to build stronger muscles and bones.

Exercise benefits

Starting a fitness regimen is never a terrible idea. Regular physical activity for postmenopausal women can:

- ➢ Increase your muscular endurance.
- ➢ Enhance your equilibrium.
- ➢ Reduce the possibility of breaking a bone.
- ➢ 'Keep or accentuate your posture.
- ➢ reduce or eliminate discomfort.

When exercising with osteoporosis, one must choose the safest, most fun activities possible for their level of bone loss and general health.

Before starting

Before beginning any fitness regimen for osteoporosis, speak with your doctor. You could initially require some tests, such as:

➢ Bone density analysis
➢ Fitness evaluation

In the meantime, think about the activities you most love doing. You're more likely to persist with a workout regimen if you choose something you enjoy doing.

Selecting the best type of exercise

People with osteoporosis are frequently advised to engage in the following activities:

➢ Exercises for building strength
➢ particularly for the upper back
➢ Aerobic exercises involving weight-bearing
➢ Flexibility training
➢ Exercises for balance and stability

You might be discouraged from doing some exercises due to the different levels of osteoporosis and the possibility of fracture. Inquire with your doctor or physical therapist about your risk of osteoporosis-related issues and what exercises would be best for you.

Strength training

All major muscle groups can be strengthened through strength training, which also includes the use of free weights, resistance bands, or your own body weight, especially the spinal muscles that are crucial for posture. Maintaining bone density can also be aided by resistance training.

Avoid twisting your spine when using weight machines, performing exercises, or making adjustments.

In particular, if you experience pain, resistance training should be customized to your level of ability and tolerance. You can create strength-training regimens with the assistance of a physical therapist or personal trainer with experience working with osteoporosis patients. In order to avoid injuries and maximize the benefits of your workout, proper form and technique are essential.

Weight-bearing aerobic activities

Aerobic exercises that involve weight bearing involve standing while carrying your weight on your bones.

Walking, dancing, low-impact aerobics, elliptical machines, stair climbing, and gardening are a few examples.

These exercises slow mineral loss by directly affecting the bones in your legs, hips, and lower spine. Additionally, they provide cardiovascular advantages that improve the condition of the heart and circulatory system.

It's crucial that aerobic exercises do not constitute your entire workout regimen, despite the fact that they are good for your general health. Additionally, it's crucial to practice balance, flexibility, and strength.

Although swimming and cycling have numerous advantages, they don't give your bones the weight-bearing load they require to reduce mineral loss. But if you like doing them, go ahead and do them. Just make sure to include as much weight-bearing exercise as you can.

Stretching exercises

Your muscles will continue to function well if you continue to move your joints through their complete range of motion. The optimal time to stretch is after your muscles have warmed up, such as at the conclusion of your workout or during a 10-minute warm-up. They ought to be carried out slowly and carefully without bouncing.

Avoid stretches that lead you to bend at the waist or flex your spine. Find out from your doctor which stretches are most effective for you.

Exercises for balance and stability

Fall prevention is crucial for those who have osteoporosis. Your muscles will cooperate in a way that makes you more stable and less likely to fall if you engage in stability and balance exercises. Your stability and balance can be improved by performing easy exercises like standing on one leg or movement-based activities like tai chi.

Exercise to avoid

If you have osteoporosis, avoid the following activities:

➢ **High-intensity exercises**

Jumping, running, or jogging can break bones that are already fragile. Always strive to avoid making sudden, swift movements. Choose exercises that call for calm, controlled movement. However, you might be able to engage in slightly more strenuous activities than someone who is frail if you are typically robust and active while having osteoporosis.

➢ **Bending and twisting.**

Exercises that require you to bend forward at the waist and twist your waist, such as doing sit-ups or touching your toes, can increase your risk of getting compression fractures in your spine if you have osteoporosis. Other pastimes that may require you to violently bend or twist your body at the waist include golf, tennis, bowling, and various yoga positions. If you're unsure of the condition of your bones, speak with your doctor. Don't let your concern about fractures keep you from enjoying yourself.

CHAPTER 6: HORMONE THERAPY

Is it appropriate for you?

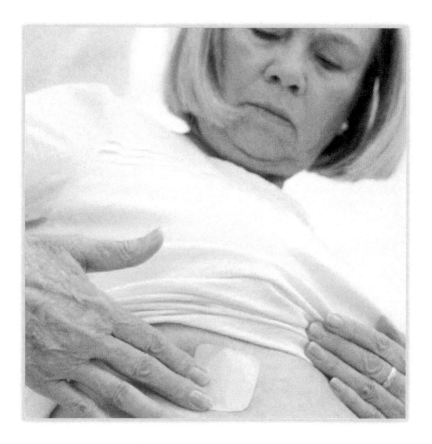

Hormone therapy was once a common treatment for menopausal symptoms and long-term health. Then, a thorough clinical study identified health risks. How does that make you feel? Medication used for hormone replacement therapy contains female hormones. The medication is taken to replace the lost estrogen brought on by menopause. Hot flashes and vaginal soreness are two common menopausal symptoms that are often treated with hormone treatment. Hormone therapy has also been demonstrated to reduce fractures and halt bone loss in postmenopausal women. Nevertheless, utilizing hormone therapy carries some hazards. These risks are influenced by the type of hormone therapy, the dosage, the length of the course, and your individual health concerns. For the greatest chance of success, hormone therapy should be tailored for each patient and often reevaluated to make sure the benefits still outweigh the drawbacks.

What are the basic types of hormone therapy?

The basic objective of hormone replacement therapy is to replace the lost estrogen that results from menopause in your body. The following are the two primary types of estrogen therapy:

➢ **Systemic hormone therapy**

Systemic estrogen, which can be used as a tablet, skin patch, ring, gel, cream, or spray and is absorbed throughout the body, frequently has a higher dose of estrogen. Any of the typical menopause symptoms can be treated with it.

➤ Low-dose vaginal products

Low-dose vaginal estrogen treatments lessen the amount of estrogen the body absorbs in the form of creams, pills, or rings. Because of this, menopausal symptoms of the urinary and vaginal systems are frequently treated using low-dose vaginal therapies.

If your uterus has not been removed, your doctor will typically prescribe estrogen along with progesterone or progestin (progesterone-like medication). This is because estrogen can promote the growth of the uterine lining on its own, raising the risk of endometrial cancer, without progesterone to balance it. If you've had a hysterectomy, it's conceivable that you won't need to take progesterone.

Which risks are associated with hormone therapy?

In hormone replacement therapy, the estrogen-progestin pill (Prempro) was found to increase the risk of various major disorders, including:

➢ heart problem
➢ Stroke
➢ clotting blood
➢ Breast cancer

The results of subsequent investigations indicate that these hazards can vary depending on:

➢ **Age**. Women who begin hormone therapy at age 60 or older or more than 10 years after menopause begins are more likely to develop the aforementioned illnesses. When hormone therapy is started before 60 or within ten years of menopause, the advantages seem to exceed the hazards.

➢ **The hormone treatment type.** The risks of hormone therapy vary according to the type and dosage of estrogen, whether it is used alone or in conjunction with progestin, and other variables.

➢ **Health background.** Your personal medical history, family history, and risk factors for cancer, heart disease, stroke, blood clots, liver disease, and osteoporosis will all play a role in determining if hormone replacement therapy is the correct choice for you.

You and your doctor should consider each of these issues before deciding whether hormone therapy is a good option for you.

Who is eligible for hormonal therapy?

If you're in good health and experience mild to severe hot flashes, the benefits of hormone therapy may outweigh the risks.

➢ Systemic estrogen therapy continues to be the most efficient treatment for troublesome menopausal hot flashes and night sweats.

➢ Additional menopausal symptoms could appear. Menopausal vaginal symptoms like dryness, itching, burning, and pain during sexual activity can be lessened with estrogen.

➢ Avoiding bone loss or fractures is essential. Systemic estrogen prevents the thinning of the bones caused by osteoporosis. But normally, doctors advise using medications called bisphosphonates to treat osteoporosis. But estrogen therapy could be able to help if other treatments aren't effective for you or you can't tolerate them. have low estrogen levels or are in early menopause.

➤ If you had your ovaries surgically removed before the age of 45, stopped receiving periods before the age of 45 (early or premature menopause), or lost normal ovarian function before the age of 40, your body has been exposed to less estrogen than the bodies of women who experience regular menopause (primary ovarian insufficiency). With the help of estrogen therapy, you can reduce your risk of developing conditions including osteoporosis, heart disease, stroke, dementia, and mood swings.

How can risk be reduced if you use hormone therapy?

Consult your doctor about the following techniques:

➤ **Find the delivery method and product that are ideal for you.** It is possible to take estrogen as a tablet, patch, gel, vaginal cream, slow-releasing suppository, or vaginal ring. A low-dose vaginal cream, tablet, or ring containing estrogen is typically preferable to an oral pill or a skin patch if all of your menopausal symptoms are vaginal.

➢ **Reduce the dosage of any medications you take**. To address your symptoms, take the smallest dose that works in the shortest amount of time. You need enough estrogen if you're under 45 to guard against the long-term negative impacts of low estrogen levels on your health. Your doctor could advise longer-term treatment if you experience persistent menopausal symptoms that significantly lower your quality of life.

➢ **Seek routine follow-up treatment.** Visit your doctor frequently to have screenings, including mammograms and pelvic exams, as well as to make sure the advantages of hormone therapy still outweigh the risks.

➢ Make wholesome lifestyle decisions. Include exercise and physical activity in your daily routine, consume a nutritious diet, keep your weight in check, abstain from alcohol and smoking, manage stress, and treat chronic health disorders like high cholesterol or high blood pressure.

You'll also require progesterone if you haven't had a hysterectomy and are taking systemic estrogen therapy. Your doctor can assist you in identifying the delivery strategy that provides the greatest convenience and advantages with the fewest risks and expenses.

If hormone therapy is not an option for you, what can you do?

Menopausal hot flashes may be controlled by healthy lifestyle practices such as maintaining a healthy body temperature, avoiding alcohol and caffeine, and engaging in paced relaxing breathing or other relaxation techniques. Additionally, a number of prescribed non-hormone drugs may reduce hot flashes.

A vaginal moisturizer or lubricant may offer treatment for vaginal issues like dryness or uncomfortable intercourse. The prescription drug ospemifene (Osphena), which may help with instances of painful intercourse, is something else you might discuss with your doctor.

The bottom line: There are both positive and harmful uses for hormone therapy.

You should discuss your unique symptoms and potential health concerns with your doctor in order to decide if hormone therapy is a good course of treatment for you. Recommendations may alter as more is discovered by researchers regarding hormone therapy and other menopausal treatments. If you experience bothersome menopausal symptoms on a regular basis, discuss treatment options with your doctor.

REFERENCES

https://www.mayoclinic.org/

https://newsnetwork.mayoclinic.org/

https://www.livestrong.com/

https://www.medicinenet.com/

https://www.healthline.com/

https://www.healthywomen.org/

Printed in Great Britain
by Amazon

22947698R00064